ELEMENTARY

PLUGGED-IN PLANNER

WRITTEN BY

Screen Sanity

IN PARTNERSHIP WITH SUSAN CROWN EXCHANGE

To order additional copies of this resource visit **screensanity.org/tools** or email at **info@screensanity.org.**

HI
THERE.

We're so glad you're here!
Before diving in, please take a moment to give yourself a pat on the back. Amidst the busyness of life, you picked up this planner and are taking action. Kudos to you! Raising kids in today's digital age is not an easy task — our children have never known a world without smartphones and social media — and this can quickly feel overwhelming. We're here to let you know that you're not alone.

There is no perfect approach to managing screens, and there will certainly be bumps along the way. However, taking time to proactively set intentions, draw boundaries, and start conversations can help to minimize the bruises and maximize the benefits.

This planner is space to help you pause and reflect at the role technology plays in your child's life. You have what it takes to help your kiddo stay **captivated by life, not screens.**

CONSIDER THE BIG PICTURE

When it comes to device introduction, three words guide our process: **"Ride. Practice. Drive."** Teaching your kid to drive a device is sort of like teaching your kid to drive a car. Similar to driver's ed, there can be an intentional process to introducing new technology.

In navigating this roadmap, it may be helpful to identify where your child is on their digital journey. Take some time to orient yourself on the following map, envisioning what your child's device use will entail in the coming years.

This will look different for every family. The end goal is not to find the magic age or correct plan, but rather to familiarize yourself with the path you plan/hope to take.

YOU ARE HERE!

RIDE	PRACTICE	DRIVE

This planner is focused on supporting parents who are in the passenger seat, helping their kids practice with devices.

RIDE

Buckle up in the back.

Start by having your child observe your digital practices and device use, similar to how we watched our parents drive from the backseat.

PRACTICE

Start small.

When it's time for a device, consider one that is simple, safe and stripped down to limited features. Allow your kid to experiment with independence and develop foundational skills. During this time, plan to log many hours riding in the passenger seat, helping them practice healthy digital habits.

DRIVE

Smartphone independence.

When he or she demonstrates competence and you feel comfortable, your child is likely ready to embark on solo device use. They'll still bump curbs or get into accidents, but they can mostly navigate sticky situations on their own.

1/

BIG DREAMS, SMALL SCREENS

From the time our children are born,
we dream about who they might become.

Will they be kind, confident and brave?

**Will they become scholars or
athletes or lawyers?**

**What will they remember from
their childhood?**

As children grow, we are lucky enough to
have a front-row seat watching them live out
their dreams. Before we dig in, let's start with
the end in mind: At the end of this parenting
journey, what will success look like?

▷|◁ **REFLECT**

Define Your Dreams

Take a moment to reflect on your dreams for your son or daughter's childhood.

What do you remember from your own childhood?

_____

_____

What are your dreams for this child?

_____

_____

How can you envision technology supporting your child in achieving their dreams? How might it get in the way?

_____

_____

When you send your child off to college, what attributes do you want them to have?

_____

_____

🔌 **PLUG IN**

Cast a Vision

Few tools are better for manifesting dreams than a good 'ole fashioned vision board. We love this fun, collaborative activity as a way to connect and share aspirations with your child.

Spread out some old magazines, grab a few supplies (scissors, glue, markers, poster board, etc.) and encourage your child to **build a collage that represents their unique goals and dreams.** Perhaps you sit alongside them and craft a vision board of your own! Hang the finished products on a wall in your home to promote motivation, focus and visualization.

2 /

SET YOUR VALUES

As the old country song goes, **"If you don't stand for something — you'll fall for anything."**

Without a plan, it's easy to get off track, especially when it comes to screen use. Think of your core values as your north star — a way to make sure your family is headed in the same direction in terms of technology and life as a whole.

What's Most Important?

Pick two to five values that you believe are important to the way you live and work as a family. Choose values that you hope your family will stick to, even in the toughest of situations.

☐ Community	☐ Integrity
☐ Connection	☐ Kindness
☐ Creativity	☐ Love
☐ Determination	☐ Productivity
☐ Empathy	☐ Recreation
☐ Encouragement	☐ Respect
☐ Exploration	☐ Self-improvement
☐ Faith	☐ Service
☐ Friendship	☐ Sustainability
☐ Giving	☐ Teamwork
☐ Grace	☐ Tolerance
☐ Gratitude	☐ Trust
☐ Hard work	☐ _____
☐ Honor	☐ _____

⚡ PLUG IN
Get in Sync

After you've had time to reflect, invite your family to join the values conversation with this simple activity.

1 **Write the above list of values on flashcards** and spread them on your kitchen table. Talk about how these values play out in the real world, as well as the digital world. Together, pick two to five values that you believe are important to the way you live and work as a family.

2 **Hang them up!** Whether you stick them on the fridge, string the cards into garland or tape them to the bathroom mirror — display them somewhere you will see them often, as a reminder of what you are striving for together.

3 **Check in regularly.** Use these values to stay in sync and start conversations about how your daily choices support your values... or get in the way of them.

Visit screensanity.org to download a printable copy of our full **Values Exercise**.

3 /

START
WITH
YOURSELF

Kids are sponges, absorbing the behaviors they see modeled in the world. **Monkey see? Monkey do!**

So, before you set out to help them develop healthy screentime habits — you must "put your oxygen mask on first."

Now, take a deep breath — this doesn't mean you have to have a perfect relationship with technology. When the rubber hits the road, your child will learn a lot more watching you navigate challenges than they would by seeing a model of perfection.

Give yourself grace and compassion as you reflect honestly on your relationship with screens.

Do a Tech Check

Our phones are a gift — but they can also interfere with the things that matter most to us. How do you feel about your relationship with your phone?

Got things
under control ①—②—③—④—⑤—⑥—⑦—⑧—⑨—⑩ Totally
overwhelmed

Describe a time when your child noticed something about your tech use.

_____

_____

There is no magic wand when it comes to finding the right screen-life balance, but small tweaks can make a world of difference in your digital health. **Check one or two steps you would like to take:**

☐ Wear a smartwatch to filter out notifications   ☐ Silence notifications

☐ Set aside your phone in times of deep focus   ☐ Remove email alerts

☐ Narrate phone activities so your kids know what you are doing
(i.e. paying bills, ordering groceries, scheduling appointments)   ☐ Delete distracting apps from your homescreen

Get Curious

Have a conversation with your child to see what they observe about your technology use. Start with something like:

"I've been thinking about my phone and how often I use it. In some ways it helps me — to connect with family, pay bills, respond to emails — but it also distracts me from what's most important. I'm curious if you've noticed anything about my phone use. What have you noticed? What would you suggest I change?"

Be open, understanding and avoid getting defensive. Let your child share truthfully about what they have witnessed. Together, pick a silly "code word" (like, "pizza") they can use in the future to let you know they need you to set your phone down and give them focused attention.

PRIORITIZE DEVICE-FREE ZONES

In 2017, the city of Boston asked all kindergarteners to design the best playground imaginable. Like the planners, you may envision twisty slides, splash pads and sand pits.

But, to their surprise, the overwhelming top request from the kindergarteners was nothing of the sorts. The main thing the kids were after?

Playgrounds that required lockers for their parents to put away their phones.

Kids already dream of the quality time brought about by device-free zones; they just need our help establishing them. If you are looking for a good place to start, we suggest tables and bedtimes.

▷|◁ **REFLECT**

Disconnect to Reconnect

When are times in the day where you have the opportunity for meaningful connection with your child?

_____

_____

Times and spaces where you hope to create device-free zones:

☐ Bedrooms   ☐ Before school/work

☐ Bathrooms   ☐ Pool/playground

☐ During meals   ☐ When friends are over

☐ Vacations   ☐ During homework

☐ In the car   ☐ _____
(except on long trips)

One of the healthiest things you can do for your child is set a norm that devices aren't in their bedroom at night. This can protect their valuable sleep. If you're interested in doing this:

Where will devices charge?   **When will devices go to sleep?**

☐ Kitchen   ☐ _____

☐ Parents' room   ☐ 1 hour before bed

☐ Home office   ☐ 8pm

☐ _____   ☐ 9pm

🔌 **PLUG IN**

Device-Free Gathering

The next time you host a gathering — a playdate, sleepover, BBQ — consider making it device-free. The secret sauce for success? **Clearly communicate on the invitation that there will be a spot for devices to be checked-in.**

You might say something like, _"We're excited to get together! Just a quick note that we're encouraging phones be set aside in a basket at the beginning of the party. If your kids need to reach you, they'll be able to come and use their phones."_

This gives parents a heads-up and prevents guests from being caught off-guard when they arrive.

5 /

BUCKLE THEIR SEATBELT

The internet can be like the classic Nintendo game Mario Kart — turtle shells and banana peels flying unexpectedly into view from every direction. While some of these hazards are harmless, others can lead to Game Over.

When your child is online, predators, bullies and porn bots can have access to them at any time. Unfortunately, there are minimal built-in safety measures, so we need to create our own precautions.

Think of these like seatbelts — offering as much protection as possible from accidents that are bound to happen in the online world.

▷|◁ REFLECT
Set Up For Safety

No solution is 100% foolproof, but there are several safety nets to help decrease risks online. Check the ones you want to employ:

- ☐ Familiarize yourself with the filters your school-issued devices use, and download the parent app if there is one
- ☐ Apply filters on home routers
- ☐ Set social accounts to private
- ☐ Turn off location on devices
- ☐ Block messages/calls from strangers
- ☐ Use Screen Sanity's "Ride. Practice. Drive." approach to introducing new devices or apps

How will you prepare your child to respond when someone asks them for personal information over a digital platform?

- ☐ Look away
- ☐ Block the person
- ☐ Close the window or toggle to the home screen
- ☐ Close the device like Pacman
- ☐ Let a trusted adult know
- ☐ _____

When your child shares — or you uncover — an awkward or shocking online situation, it's critical you don't overreact. Pick a phrase you want to practice to ensure you keep your "poker face." Below are some thought-starters:

- ☐ Tell me more.
- ☐ Thanks so much for trusting me with this.
- ☐ Gosh, that's interesting. How did that make you feel?
- ☐ I'd love to hear more. Want to grab some ice cream and chat?
- ☐ I'm so glad you know you can tell me anything. I am always here.

Pick a code word you can establish with your kids so they feel equipped when they see something inappropriate and need to talk:

_____

⚡ PLUG IN
Have the Talk

Starting a conversation about hazards like pornography and online predators is easier said than done — but, we promise, there is hope. We recommend reading the book *Good Pictures Bad Pictures* with your child. The internationally acclaimed, read-aloud story features a mom and dad who explain what pornography is, why it's dangerous and how to reject it. We've found it to be gentle and effective in introducing conversations about the topic in a safe, straight-forward way.

CHAPTER SIX

RHYTHMS ARE YOUR FRIEND

Creating boundaries, or a rhythm with your time on screens, is not for the faint of heart. This is tough work, especially at the beginning. But, when consistency is held, the predicable patterns will take the fall for being the bad guy and you will be let off the hook. **You'll fight less battles as your kids know what to expect and that you hold true to your word.**

Make A Mantra

Take a moment and brainstorm a technology rhythm that can become your family's mantra. Don't stress about how other families do it — just create something attainable that supports your family's unique needs. Here are a couple of examples to use as inspiration — or create your own!

(1)   Braintime. Chores. Screens. Outdoors.

(2)   No screens before noon.

(3)   Phone put up. Teeth brushed. Books read. Time for bed.

(4)   Good night, screens. Hello, sweet dreams.

Consider striving for a 1:1 online to offline ratio. For every half hour spent engaged with screens, we encourage a half hour spent engaged with real life. Or, perhaps you call this your Rule of 30: For every 30 minutes of time with tech, you have 30 minutes of unplugged time.

Feeling inspired? Brainstorm some mantras of your own:

_____

_____

Reveal the Roadmap

Kids know the power of these five words: "But everyone else has one!" However, when it comes to devices, your child is likely not the only one left emptyhanded. The trend is heading in a new direction, with a growing number of parents delaying smartphone introduction. The right time is different for every family, but by **establishing expectations early (about when your child will get a phone or device), you'll help prevent future meltdowns.** Cast a vision for your child by saying something like,

"I know you asked about getting your own phone and I have good news: you will get a smartphone someday! When you are old enough to need a way to call me, (maybe in __ grade), we'll start with a first phone that will help you learn the ropes. I'm excited for how this device is going to give you more freedom and how you're going to be able to keep in touch with some of your friends. As you demonstrate skills, showing you're ready to have more, we'll add on new layers, and I'll be celebrating that growth alongside you!"

AVOIDING MELTDOWNS

As adults, our brains are tasked with the job of scrolling, sifting and responding to a world of digital noise — overflowing inboxes, nonstop notifications, social media interactions.

But when our children spend time immersed in apps and devices, their developing brains can't always keep up with the stimulation.

The pre-frontal cortex is the part of the brain responsible for decision-making, higher reasoning, judgment and self-control — and it won't be in place until age 25!

In the meantime, kids need your loving support to help them identify their personal limits, and learn to log off screens before a meltdown occurs.

See the Change

The number one indicator that your child's brain has reached its limit is behavior change. When you notice this happening, it's a sign they'll need your help in coregulating their emotions and decision-making.

When do you find it most difficult to transition off screens without a meltdown? Can you identify "early indicators" that a meltdown is coming?

_____

_____

What are some things you might try to help your child learn to transition off screens without a meltdown?

- ☐ Touch them on the shoulder
- ☐ Allow them to finish the level they have been working on
- ☐ Use calm language like, "Find a good place to stop."
- ☐ Sit down next to them and help them stop the show or game
- ☐ Help them learn to monitor their own tech time minutes
- ☐ Help them set their own timer for video games or shows
- ☐ Teach them the "tricks" tech companies use to keep them glued to their screens
- ☐ Narrate your own transitions out loud to model a healthy approach

What activities best help your child reset after they log off?

- ☐ Going outside
- ☐ Helping prep dinner
- ☐ Performing household chores
- ☐ Walking the dog
- ☐ Going to the library
- ☐ Doing creative projects
- ☐ Journaling
- ☐ _____

Find Your Flow

A resource to support you in coregulation is our **Video Game Decision Tree.** This flowchart helps families get on the same page about time limits. Visit screensanity.org to download a printable copy to share with your kids. Perhaps you even hang it near the gaming station as a reminder of what you're striving for! Remember that decision-making and emotional regulation are skills your kiddo is still developing. It may take a few tries before you find their goldilocks "just right" limit.

8 /

QUALITY VS. QUANTITY

The digital world wants to keep you scrolling, but at the end of life, all you have is your time and attention.

When you look back, what will you (and your child) say was time well spent?

What if instead of a platform for endless consumption, screens were intentionally used to spark creation?

One of the most forward-thinking things we can do as parents is to team up with technology, helping our kids see it as a means to an end — a mode for driving creativity, curiosity and connection — and not the goal itself.

▷|◁ **REFLECT**

Plug In With Purpose

What are ways your child enjoys being creative or things your child likes to create? Are they an expert in paper airplanes, a fashion connoisseur in coordinating outfits or a master doodler? Do they prepare gourmet snacks or build elaborate Lego formations? How do they enjoy engaging with the world around them?

_____

_____

_____

_____

Is there any opportunity of overlap between your child's passions and their use of technology? Jot down a few ways that their plugged-in time can become more purposeful:

_____

_____

⚡ **PLUG IN**

Create More Than You Consume

Take some time to reflect on how you liked to play as a child and see if you can recapture that creativity in your digital world. Maybe this is researching and reading about something you're passionate about, finding an artist app or learning a new language. Or, maybe it's using your social media as creative writing outlet instead of a scroll fest.

Once you've experimented with this concept, invite your kiddo to join you in **engaging with technology in a higher quality way.** Look up complex paper airplane patterns to build and then test which ones best take flight, learn phrases in a different language together, or help them research their favorite animal. The possibilities are endless.

For more ideas, download our **30 Days of Creation** _PDF at screensanity.org._

FIND YOUR VILLAGE

Raising kids in the digital world is hard, but it's even harder to do it alone. One of the best ways you can stay in the game is finding other parents to link arms with when it comes to technology boundaries. It can be overwhelming to start a conversation with other parents — but the sooner you start, the more you will benefit and "get ahead" of the challenges to come.

▷|◁ **REFLECT**

Start a Convo

Is there someone you feel safe talking to as you navigate the challenges of raising kids in a digital world?

_____

_____

Is there someone who you need to communicate your boundaries or concerns surrounding screens with? What are your hesitations — and what is the best possible outcome from?

_____

_____

Describe your vision for what it looks like to have a community of people who are on the same page when it comes to digital health. What can you do to help support your community in this challenging issue?

_____

_____

⚡ **PLUG IN**

Gather a Group

As parents, we share everything from our favorite recipes to the best neighborhood babysitters. But when it comes to raising kids in the digital world, we often feel as if we're navigating an unpaved road alone. We believe there is power community, in having a group of parents who can gather together, have each other's backs and discover solutions to shared screentime struggles.

The Screen Sanity Group Study allows you to do just that. This interactive handbook features a collection of video-guided sessions that cover every age and stage of digital childhood – from tech use to smartphone introduction. It was designed to spark face-to-face conversations with others in a casual setting.

The Group Study can take place in a variety of contexts: around a kitchen table with your book club, in the school library with your PTO, or on the driveway with neighbors as the kids ride bikes down the street. Visit screensanity.org for more details on starting a Screen Sanity Group Study.

You were never meant to do parenthood alone...let's continue this journey together!

Screen Sanity is here for you at each milestone and tech-related challenge.

Continue to stay "plugged in" with our next book,
Plugged-in Planner: Middle School.

SCREENSANITY.ORG

Notes

www.ingramcontent.com/pod-product-compliance
Lightning Source LLC
Chambersburg PA
CBHW041106050426

42335CB00047B/171